GOUT HATER'S

COOKBOOK IV

THE LOW PURINE DIET COOKBOOK

JODI HOCKINSON
DTR/NDTR, CDM, CFPP

Gout Hater's Cookbook IV
The low purine diet cookbook
ISBN 10: 1-888141-77-8
ISBN13: 978-1-888141-77-1

Please note: The contents of this book are in no way intended for use as a substitute for medical advice. Always consult your physician before making any changes in your diet. The information provided may vary from the regimen given to you by your physician or dietitian. As every individual case is different, please follow your recommended regimen, including exercise, diet and medications.

Published by
Southeast Media Productions
Carlisle, PA
USA |
Phone: 386-503-6832
www.gout-haters.com

Many thanks to the Purine Research Society and its efforts to help children with purine autism.

Table of Contents

A Little About Gout Hater's Cookbook IV

When the original *Gout Hater's Cookbook* was published more than 10 years ago, only 1.2 million people in the United States suffered from gout. Today, the number is many times that amount, at 8.3 million, and growing.

Research for the first book was frustrating, as there were not many publications concerning gout and diet, and the few publications that existed tended to contradict each other continually.

Indeed, there are still quite a few controversies concerning what can and cannot be tolerated, and whether a low-purine diet should be recommended. Many physicians feel that placing a patient on restriction can lead to binges on the very foods that should be avoided. In this spirit, the *Gout Hater's Cookbook* series has strived to demonstrate precisely how wonderfully tasty a diet can be, especially when focus is placed on the foods that are included in the diet, rather than the foods that are restricted.

In fact, when one third of the uric acid level is normally affected by diet, watching what you eat can make a crucial difference in your well being.

Gout Hater's Cookbook IV has been presented in celebration of that positive way of thinking: focus on what you can have and forget about the rest!

With new research results being reported, we have been able to add some things that were not previously available in the *Gout Hater's Cookbook* series, as well as report updates that we have found.

Although all books in the *Gout Hater's* collection are continuously revised, it has been exciting to present all-new recipes with ingredients that we have not been able to use before!

For example, long-term research reports state that high purine vegetables (although moderate use is recommended) do not increase the risk of gout (please see "Important Research Results" for more details).

In addition, meat recipes have been included in this volume, but only to be used with physician's approval (Please see "About Meat Recipes").

Book IV also contains a master index of all four *Gout Hater's Cookbooks*. Although each volume is designed to be used independently of the others, *Gout Hater's* readers have been requesting an index that will allow them to quickly figure out which volume contains a favorite recipe.

What is Gout?

Gout is a condition that is brought on as a result of the inability for the body to eliminate uric acid, a naturally occurring chemical.

About one third of the body's uric acid normally comes from diet, and is a by-product of purines. As the level of uric acid in the blood increases, it becomes less soluble. Too much uric acid in the blood is known as hyperurecemia. the solubility of uric acid can be affected by pH level as well as differences in temperature. This explains why attacks of gout usually occur in the body's extremities, such as the big toe, where the temperature is likely to be lower.

Needle-like crystals, called tophi, will form around connective tissue or joint spaces, causing inflammation that can be so painful that even the weight of a bed sheet can inflict excruciating pain.

There are many contributors that can cause an attack of gout, even overnight, including dehydration and excessive alcohol consumption. Other risk factors include renal insufficiency, use of salicylates (including aspirin), consumption of high purine foods, hypertension, use of diuretics, obesity, extreme changes in diet, surgery and trauma.

More than 8.3 million people in the United States suffer from gout. This represents an increase of about seven times the 1.2 million that were affected when the original *Gout Hater's Cookbook* became available.

Most are men over the age of 40; a small percentage are women, usually after reaching menopause.

Treatment of gout can include pain relieving and preventive medications, reduced alcohol consumption and a diet of low purine foods. Indeed, gout is said to be the only rheumatic disease that can be substantially affected by diet.

Important Research Results

According to a twelve-year study published in the New England Journal of Medicine, it is no longer necessary to avoid vegetables that are high in purines. However, the study recommends a moderate consumption of these foods, stating there is no association between a moderate intake and the risk of out.

In addition, a daily intake of low-fat or non-fat milk and yogurt was seen to reduce the risk of gout.

In contrast, one serving of meat per day increased the risk by 21%, and one serving of fish per week, increased the risk by 7%. This means that three servings of fish per week increased the risk of gout by as much as seven servings of meat (at one per day). According to these figures, one serving of fish is more than twice as dangerous as one serving of meat!

Another interesting development published in June of 2007 was a study indicating that increased coffee consumption over a long term may not be beneficial, and could ultimately contribute to an increase in the risk of gout.

Coffee contains the antioxidant phenol chlorogenic acid, which is believed to help in insulin sensitivity. On the other hand, although caffeine may act as a xanthine oxidase inhibitor (as is allopurinol, blocking the metabolizing of purines into uric acid), it also acts to *lower* insulin sensitivity, which could ultimately cause an increase in the risk of gout.

Therefore, it cannot be stressed enough that your diet should adhere to the recommendations of your physician, and many factors can be involved in what is set forth in your regimen.

FOODS ALLOWED
- GREEN LIGHT -
LOWEST LEVEL PURINES

Beets (except beet tops), berries, broccoli, carrots, celery, coconuts, corn, cucumbers, fruits and fruit juice, eggplant, green string beans (not bulging), grits, hominy, jicama, leafy greens (except those listed in the moderate level group), leeks, lettuce, okra, olives, onions, parsnips, peppers, potatoes, radishes, rhubarb, sago, squash, tomatoes, turnips, vegetables soups (not containing meat stock, meat extracts or high-purine vegetables), water chestnuts

Nuts (except peanuts - see "Legumes and Complete Proteins")

Dairy (low fat or fat free): cottage cheese, cheese, eggs (nor more than yolk per day; more than one white is allowed), ice cream, margarine, milk, ricotta, yogurt. Watch the ingredients for xanthan/xanthum gum or xanthene.

Cereals (except whole grain); corn flakes, semolina pasta/macaroni (preferably 100% semolina), white rice, tapioca

White flour (without malted barley flour added), matzoh, white rice flour, arrowroot flour, baker's yeast (only as a part of baking. Yeast supplements are not allowed), white bread, French bread, plain white bagels (watch for malt). white pita bread

Ketchup, mustard, mayonnaise, honey, sugar

Decaf coffee, tea, sodas: non-cola, non-caffeine

Vegetable oils: canola, olive soy

FOODS ALLOWED
- YELLOW LIGHT -
MODERATE LEVEL PURINES

The following non-meat items are allowed, but are grouped differently here only because they contain higher purine levels. According to a 12-year study published in the New England Journal of Medicine, a moderate amount of vegetables rich in purines did not increase the risk of gout.

Artichokes, asparagus, beans, bean sprouts, beet tops, bok choy, Brussels sprouts, cabbage, cauliflower, dried beans and peas, kale, legumes, lentils, mushrooms, peanuts and peanut butter, peanut oil, peas, soy/soy products (including tofu, soy sauce and soy flour), spinach, Swiss chard

Wheat germ and whole grain cereal or flour, including barley, barley malt, bran, brown rice, oatmeal, oats, rye, pumpernickel, graham flour, malt, whole wheat, whole wheat flour; macaroni products not labeled as semolina or durum semolina

Your system may be able to tolerate 3 ounces (about the size of a deck of cards) of the following foods per day (Please check with your physician or dietitian):

Skinless white meat chicken or turkey

Beef: Your prescribed diet may also allow small servings of beef (included in Foods not Allowed). Therefore, a small number of recipes that contain reduced serving sizes of meat have been provided.

FOODS AND INGREDIENTS NOT ALLOWED
- RED LIGHT -
AVOID THESE ITEMS

The following foods and ingredients are either very high in purines or otherwise not allowed in the restricted purine diet (See "Important Research Results").

Alcoholic beverages, coffee, chocolate, cocoa, cola drinks, carob, carob bean gum, caffeine.

All types of seafood, especially anchovies, caviar, fish roe, herring, ocean perch, sardines, scallops, smelt, sprat, trout and tuna.

The following meats are very high in purines: game meats, horse, kidney, lamb, meat extracts, muscle, organ meats, sausage, spleen and tongue.

The following meats are *only relatively high* in purines, but not recommended, because they are high in saturated fats: beef (brisket, chuck, filet, shoulder, rump, corned beef), dark meat chicken or poultry and poultry skin, pork (bacon, chop, chuck, filet, hind leg, shoulder), meat broth, veal filet or shoulder.

Brewer's yeast, yeast supplements, seeds, MSG, xanthine, xanthan/xanthum gum, lard, powdered or evaporated milk, whole milk/whole milk products.

Salicylates

The following list shows some examples of salicylates, which should be avoided. Salicylates can worsen your condition as well as adversely affect the potency of some medications.

Acuprin 81

Amigesic

Anacin Caplets

Anacin Maximum Strength

Anacin Tablets

Anaflex 750

Arthritis Pain Ascriptin

Arthritis Pain Formula

Arthritis Strength Bufferin

Arthropan

Aspergum

Aspirin Regimen Bayer Adult Low Dose

Aspirin Regimen Bayer Regular Strength Caplets

Aspir-Low

Aspirtab

Aspirtab-Max

Backache Caplets

Empirin

Extended-Release Bayer 8-Hour

Extra Strength Bayer Arthritis Pain Formula Caplets

Extra Strength Bayer Aspirin Caplets

Extra Strength Bayer Aspirin Tablets

Extra Strength Bayer Plus Caplets

Gensan

Genuine Bayer Aspirin Caplets

Genuine Bayer Aspirin Tablets

Halfprin

Healthprin Adult Low Strength

Healthprin Full Strength

Bayer Children's Aspirin

Bayer Select Maximum Strength Backache Pain Relief Formula

Bufferin Caplets

Bufferin Tablets

Buffex

Buffinol

Buffinol Extra

Cama Arthristis Pain Reliever

CMT

Cope

Disalcid

Doan's Regular Strength Tablets

Easprin

Ecotrin Caplets

Ecotrin Tablets

Healthprin Half-Dose

Magan

Magnaprin

Marthritic

Maximum Strength Arthritis Foundation Safety Coated Aspirin

Maximum Strength Ascriptin

Maximum Strength Doan's Analgesic Caplets

Mobidin

Mono-Gesic

Norwich Aspirin

P-A-C Revised Formula

Regular Strength Ascriptin

Salflex

Salsitab

Sloprin

St. Joseph Adult Chewable Aspirin

Tricosal

Trilisate

ZORprin

A more comprehensive list may be obtained from your physician or local pharmacist.

METRIC CONVERSION CHART

Weight

1 pound (lb.) = 0.4536 kg

1 ounce (weighed) = 28.35 g

Volume

1 cup = 0.2365 liter

2 cups (1 pint) = 0.473 liter

4 cups (1 quart) = 0.946 liter

4 quarts (1 gallon) = 3.784 liters

1 teaspoon = 5 ml

1 Tablespoon = 15 ml

1 ounce (⅛ cup - volume) = 30 ml

CONVERTING
FAHRENHEIT TO CELSIUS

All of the cooking temperatures used in the *Gout Hater's Cookbook* series are shown in degrees Fahrenheit. Degrees Fahrenheit can be converted to degrees Celsius as follows:

1. Begin with degrees Fahrenheit

2. Subtract 32

3. Multiply by 5

4. Divide by 9

USING RAW INGREDIENTS VS. MSG

MSG, or monosodium glutamate, contains two forms of glutamic acid: one which occurs naturally in raw ingredients, and one which is manufactured or processed.

The naturally occurring form of glutamic acid has not been found to cause adverse reactions in humans.

However, the manufactured or processed form of glutamic acid, an excitotoxin, has been reported to cause a great number of harmful effects, such as seizures, severe asthma attacks and heart arrhythmia, to name a few.

In fact, laboratory animals tested with processed or manufactured free glutamic acid developed retinal damage and brain lesions.

The GDA currently does not require "MSG" or "monosodium glutamate" to be listed in product ingredients unless it has been added separately.

Therefore, a product containing a significant amount of MSG may actually not have it listed as an ingredient. For example, hydrolyzed vegetable protein contains up to 40% MSG.

indeed, both hydrolyzed vegetable and animal protein are considered natural ingredients, as they originate from natural sources, such as pork blood, which is placed through a fermentation process.

Adding to the confusion on product labeling, descriptions such as "spices," natural flavor" or simply, "flavor," can legally be used as a description of hydrolyzed protein, which contains MSG. Interestingly, these descriptions, such as "spices," could also be referring to ingredients that contain no MSG, or a combination of the two!

Unfortunately, the ambiguity in labeling can deprive a conscientious shopper from effectively determining the MSG content of a product when looking at the label.

Therefore, it seems that the only defense against ingesting MSG is to use as many raw ingredients in the kitchen as possible. Avoid pre-packaged foods, such as sauce mixes, boxed dinners, and any items that show ingredients besides the essentials.

Sometimes the generic brand of a product will contain fewer added ingredients, especially concerning dairy products.

Be wary of products that say "No MSG Added." This indicates that the separate ingredient was not individually added, but the product might include ingredients that contain MSG.

Moreover, the artificial sweetener aspartame also is an excitotoxin that has been reported to cause identical ill effects to those reacting from MSG. Therefore, there are no recipes contained in this book that contain artificial sweeteners.

Following is a list of product ingredients that always contain MSG:

calcium caseinate

gelatin

glutamate

glutamic acid

hydrolyzed corn gluten

hydrolyzed vegetable or animal protein

monosodium glutamate

monopotassium glutamate

natrium glutamate

textured protein

yeast extract

yeast food

yeast nutrient

Ingredients that Often Contain MSG:

barley malt

bouillon

carrageenan

citric acid

corn syrup

cornstarch

enzymes/enzyme modified gums

fermented

flavor(s) or flavoring

protease/protease enzymes

protein fortified

seasonings

soy protein/soy protein concentrate or isolate

soy sauce/soy sauce extract

spices

stock

ultra-pasteurized

wheat/rice/oat protein

whey protein/whey protein concentrate or isolate

yeast nutrients

MENU SUGGESTIONS

Recipes for Autumn and Winter

Appetizers:

Baked Cheese Rolls

Cheese Balls

Baked Corn-Pepper Fritters

Hot and Sour Soup

Tomato Bisque

Corn and Okra Chowder

Spiced Buttermilk

Main Dishes:

Baked Zucchini

Baked Squash

Veggie Gumbo

Rice Chili

Eggplant Casserole

Baked Rosemary Shells

Baked Spinach

Chicken and Dressing Casserole

Chicken Curry

Chicken and Dumplings

Sides:

Almond bread

Yorkshire Pudding Puffs

Browned Onions

Labni Cheese Salad

Red Cabbage

Baked Okra

Creamed Spinach

Desserts:

Gingerbread Cake

Almond Cookies

Yogurt Cheesecake

Twice Baked Sweet Potatoes

Cherry Crepes

Recipes for Summer and Spring

Appetizers:

BBQ Broiled Tofu

Pickled Peppers

Marinated Tofu Blocks

Vichyssoise

Grilled Veggie Kabobs

Pineapple Yogurt Shake

Homemade Cherry Soda

Main Dishes:

Rice Parmesan

Eggplant Pizza

Tofu and Veggie Casserole

Egg and Macaroni Salad

Garden Pasta

Green Bean Casserole

Linguine Pesto

Broccoli Casserole

Pineapple Chicken

Chicken Kabob

Baked Chicken Dijon

Sweet Barbeque Chicken

Chicken Salad

Sides:

Coleslaw

Dijon Pasta Salad

Waldorf Salad

Feta Cheese Salad

Mozzarella Salad

Sweet Jicama Salad

Desserts:

Cheesecake Chiffon pie

Apple Pie

Carrot Cake

Cherry Cheese Cake

Lemon Pudding

PRESENTATION

Don't forget that the inviting, pleasant look of a dish can be the majority of the battle when adapting to changes in your diet. make sure that the preparation you are serving looks attractive and worth the effort.

Have you noticed that gourmet restaurants will spend a great deal of time on the look of the dish in addition to the preparation itself? For example, a plain tray of apple slices can be transformed into a welcome treat when arranged in a simple pattern, and it takes just a few more seconds to accomplish.

LEGUMES
AND
COMPLETE PROTEINS

Although legumes are relatively high in purines, a long-term study has shown that moderate intake does not increase the risk of gout (Please see "Important Research Results"). With the exception of soy, legumes contain incomplete proteins and should be eaten together with grains, effectively completing a protein balance. the two combined are "complementary proteins." Examples of a complementary protein serving include: beans with rice, bread with peanut butter and corn with peas.

Examples of the various grains that may be used with legumes to make a complementary protein are corn, pasta, bread, macaroni, rice and couscous. Quinoa is considered a complete protein.

Following are some examples of legumes:

adzuki beans

black beans

black-eyed peas (cowpeas, black-eyed beans)

butter beans

cannellini

Chickpeas (garbanzo beans)

cranberry beans (not to be confused with cranberries)

fava beans (broad beans)

flageolets

great northern beans

kidney beans

lentils

lima beans

mung beans

navy beans

peanuts

peas

pinto beans

red beans

soy beans

spit peas

white beans

ADDITIONAL NOTES

The pH level in your blood can make a huge difference in the solubility of uric acid and reduction in the risk of gout. The higher the acidity, the less soluble the uric acid. Eating foods that help balance the pH level can make a big difference.

Interestingly, some foods that are very acidic actually turn alkaline during the digestion process. For example, lemon juice is quite acidic, but the alkaline ash produced in digestion helps level the pH balance.

Vinegar is usually acid forming in the body; however, apple cider vinegar is an exception: although apple cider vinegar is acidic going in, it produces an alkaline ash upon digestion and actually helps reduce acidity.

Other examples of alkaline forming foods are orange and tomato juice. Sugar and artificial sweeteners are acid forming. remember to consume desserts only in moderation.

Vitamin C can help reduce uric acid levels. A clinical study showed that 500 mg of Vitamin C per day for 2 months reduced the serum uric acid level by .5mg per dl.

About one third of the uric acid normally produced in the body comes from food, with the remainder being produced through regular metabolism.

A daily intake of at least ½ pound of cherries has been said to help reduce uric acid levels in some cases.

Consuming meat increases the risk of gout!!! However, your physician may feel as though your system can safely tolerate skinless, white meat chicken or turkey. In some cases, of your physician has allowed you to consume a small amount of beef, please be sure to boil your meat at some point in preparation. Discard the broth!

This will help reduce the total amount of purines consumed. In this spirit, there have been several meat recipes included in this book. Although these recipes provide preparation forms that will help reduce the amount of intake and/or the amount of purines, they should be used only with the approval of your physician. Please note that beef remains on the "Foods and Ingredients not Allowed" list.

Add salt in food preparations, not at the table. In addition, try substituting half of the salt in a recipe with garlic powder or fresh minced garlic. be sure that your food is seasoned to taste before it reaches the table. This will help in lessening the total salt amount of the dinner plate.

When choosing dairy products, select low-fat or non-fat, but watch for xanthine, xanthum/xanthan gum or unspecified gums. Xanthine, a purine base, appears in the metabolism of purines to uric acid. Xanthan gum, not to be confused with xanthine (similar root sound), was tested and found to be very high in purines.

Avoid saturated fats! There are a number of beef, pork and veal cuts that are only relatively high in purines, but they can contain a great deal of saturated fat. please remember that consuming any meat or seafood servings can increase the risk of gout!

Salicylates (including aspiring) are not allowed. Please see "Salicylates" for a list of examples. Salicylates can worsen your condition or affect the potency of other medications.

Eggs should be limited to one yolk per day. More than one white is acceptable. This primarily due to the cholesterol content.

Water: Try to drink eight to ten 8-ounce glasses of water each day. Water can help flush uric acid from the system and fight against dehydration, a risk factor for gout.

Avoid extreme changes in diet, especially during an attack of gout. Moderation is the key in your dieting habits; always make any changes gradually.

Alcohol and nicotine: Not only can excessive alcohol consumption trigger an attack of gout, alcohol can inhibit the effects of medications, including allopurinol!

Nicotine intake can be a major factor in the causes of gout. If you are a smoker, try to reduce your intake. Nicotine affects blood pressure, the central nervous system, heartbeat and breathing rates, which can all add up to an increased risk for gout. In addition, when nicotine is used in conjunction with alcohol, the amount of addiction is said to increase.

BREAKFAST

Cherry Muffins

2 cups flour

1 teaspoon salt

1¾ teaspoons baking powder

¼ cup sugar

2 egg whites

1 cup skim milk

⅛ cup canola oil

½ teaspoon vanilla extract

1 cup fresh cherries, pitted and chopped

Line muffin pan with paper muffin liners, or lightly coat with margarine. Set aside.

Combine all ingredients except cherries. Blend with an electric mixer until smooth. Fold in cherries. Fill each liner ⅔ full with batter.

Bake at 350 degrees for about 20 minutes, or until a toothpick inserted in the center comes out clean. Cool and serve. makes about one dozen.

Variations: Use fresh whole blueberries. Use fresh pitted whole cherries

The fresh cherries can also be substituted with canned, drained cherries.

Sour Cream Coffee Cake

¼ cup crushed corn flakes

2 teaspoons cinnamon

¼ cup brown sugar

½ cup canola oil

1 cup sugar

3 egg whites

1 cup fat free sour cream

1 teaspoon salt

1½ cups flour

1¾ teaspoons baking powder

1 teaspoon vanilla

Preheat oven to 350 degrees. Lightly coat a Bundt pan with margarine or canola oil. Set aside. Combine corn flakes, cinnamon and brown sugar in a bowl. blend well and set aside.

Combine remaining ingredients in a large mixing bowl. blend with an electric mixer until smooth. pour one half of batter into Bundt pan.

Sprinkle one half of corn flakes mixture evenly over batter. Pour in remaining batter.

Sprinkle remaining corn flakes mixture evenly over batter.

Bake at 350 degrees for 45 minutes, or until a toothpick inserted halfway between center and wall of Bundt pan comes out clean.

Cool, turn over and serve. Serves 8.

Western Quiche

one 9-inch pie shell recipe, uncooked (see recipe)

¾ cup Swiss cheese, grated

¾ cup Colby cheese, grated

¼ cup diced green bell peppers

¼ cup diced onions

¼ cup diced red bell peppers

1 cup skim milk

]2 teaspoons flour

3 eggs

Preheat oven to 350 degrees.

Sprinkle cheese, bell peppers and onions evenly in pie shell. Set aside.

Combine milk, flour and eggs in a small mixing bowl. Blend well with a whisk or electric mixer. pour evenly over ingredients in pie shell. Bake at 350 degrees or until a knife inserted in the center comes out clean.

Allow to cool at least 10 minutes before serving.

Peasant Cheese Casserole

4 slices of cubed French bread (stale is best

1½ cups gruyere cheese, grated

4 eggs

1½ cups skim milk

1½ teaspoons mustard

1 teaspoon salt

Preheat oven to 350 degrees.

Lightly coat a 2-quart casserole dish with margarine or canola oil. Place bread in casserole dish. top with cheese. Set aside.

Combine remaining ingredients in a medium mixing bowl. Blend with a whisk until smooth.

Pour gently into casserole dish. Gently press down any bread that is not covered by the milk mixture.

Bake at 350 degrees for 45 minutes. Allow to cool 10 minutes before serving. Serve hot or warm. Serves 4 to 6.

Applesauce Cake

1¼ cups applesauce

¼ cup margarine

1¾ cups flour

½ teaspoon salt

1 teaspoon baking soda

¾ cup brown sugar

¾ teaspoon cinnamon

½ teaspoon ground cloves

¼ teaspoon allspice

2 eggs

1 cup raisins

Preheat oven to 350 degrees. Lightly coat an 8 x 8 inch pan with margarine. Set aside.

Combine all ingredients, except raisins, in a large mixing bowl. Blend with an electric mixer until smooth.

Fold in raisins. Transfer to pan. Bake for 30 minutes at 350 degrees, or until a toothpick inserted in the center comes out clean. Serves 6-8.

Cheese Grits

½ cup grits

1½ cups water

¼ teaspoon salt

2 ounces grated cheese

Combine grits, water and salt. Bring to a boil, reduce heat and simmer, stirring often, until desired consistency is reached. Fold in cheese and serve. Serves 2.

Apple Pancakes

one apple

1 teaspoon lemon juice

2 Tablespoons brown sugar

⅛ teaspoon cinnamon

batter from one recipe **fluffy pancakes**

powdered sugar

Peel, core and chop apple into small pieces. Combine with lemon juice, sugar and cinnamon. Cook in a small saucepan, stirring often, for 3-4 minutes, or until liquid is reduced and apples become a desired consistency. Allow to cool for at least 5 minutes.

Prepare fluffy pancake batter according to instructions. Fold in apples and cook as directed in pancake recipe. Serve sprinkled with powdered sugar. Makes one dozen.

Fluffy Pancakes

1 egg

3 Tablespoons margarine, softened

1 cup skim milk

¾ teaspoon salt

1¾ teaspoons baking powder

1¼ cups flour

Separate egg. Beat white with an electric mixer until stiff. Set aside.

Combine remaining ingredients in medium mixing bowl. Blend with electric mixer until smooth.

Fold in egg whites. Pour, in 4-inch circles, into a pre-heated non-stick skillet.

Cook until the surface begins to bubble and slightly dry, and the bottom lightly browns, then flip and cook until lightly browned.

Makes 10-12 pancakes.

Cherry Preserves

2 pounds fresh cherries

1½ pounds sugar

3 Tablespoons lemon juice

Remove pits from cherries, leaving them as whole as possible. Reserve any juice that comes from pitting the cherries.

Place cherries and juice along with sugar in a large pot.

Cook over low heat until the sugar dissolves, then bring slowly to a boil, stirring often.

Continue cooking at a gentle boil, stirring often, until a thick syrup forms.

Add the lemon juice and continue boiling for about 5 minutes, stirring often, until the syrup begins to set.

Pour into 12-ounce mason jars, cool, cover and refrigerate. Makes about 24 ounces of preserves.

APPETIZERS AND BEVERAGES

Baked Cheese Rolls

½ cup ricotta cheese

1 egg

¾ cup flour

¼ cup skim milk

1 teaspoon dried parsley

¼ teaspoon oregano

½ teaspoon salt

Preheat oven to 350 degrees. Lightly coat a cooking tray with olive oil. Set aside.

Combine ingredients in a medium mixing bowl. Blend well. Drop by teaspoonfuls onto cooking tray.

Bake at 350 degrees for 20 minutes. Serve with olive oil for dipping. Makes 1½ dozen.

BBQ Broiled Tofu

12 blocks of tofu, ½" x 1" x 2"

one recipe barbeque sauce (see recipe)

Lightly coat a cookie sheet with canola oil. Brush both sides of tofu blocks with barbeque sauce. Place on cookie sheet and broil at 400 degrees 4-6 minutes per side, or 350 degrees 10 minutes per side.

Brush once more with barbeque sauce and serve. Makes 12.

Pickled Peppers

4 bell peppers

1 minced onion

6 sprigs fresh dill weed, chopped

3 cups apple cider vinegar

½ cup sugar

¼ teaspoon salt

2 one-quart mason jars

Wash and remove pith from bell peppers. Cut into bite size pieces. Place one half in each of the two mason jars.

Top with one half of onion and half of the dill weed in each jar. Set aside.

Bring vinegar, sugar and salt to a boil, stirring occasionally. Allow to cool, then pour one half each over ingredients in the mason jars.

Seal and refrigerate for at least two weeks. Scrumptious!

Cheese Balls

8 ounces low fat cream cheese

1 Tablespoon flour

¼ teaspoon salt

¼ cup grated parmesan cheese

¼ teaspoon oregano

one half recipe Italian bread crumbs (see recipe)

Combine all ingredients, except bread crumbs, in a medium mixing bowl. Blend with an electric mixer until all is evenly distributed. Toll into 1-inch balls. roll balls in bread crumbs. makes about 1½ dozen.

Baked Corn-Pepper Fritters

2 cups water

1¾ cups cornmeal

½ cup chopped chili peppers or jalapeños

6 Tablespoons margarine, softened

3 teaspoons salt

1¾ teaspoons baking powder

1 egg

3½ cups flour

Preheat oven to 350 degrees. Lightly coat a cooking tray with margarine or canola oil.

Combine ingredients in a large mixing bowl. Blend until all is evenly distributed.

Drop by heaping teaspoonfuls onto cooking tray. Bake at 350 degrees for 30 minutes.

Open one to check for doneness. makes about 3 dozen.

Hot and Sour Soup

3 cups vegetable bouillon (see recipe)

2 Tablespoons apple cider vinegar

6 green onions, finely chopped

½ teaspoon salt

¼ teaspoon pepper

1 egg

1 cup extra firm tofu, cubed

Combine all ingredients, except tofu and egg, in a large saucepan. Bring to a boil. Reduce heat to a simmer.

In a small mixing bowl, beat egg with a whisk. Drop into simmering soup.

Allow egg to cook. Add tofu. Continue to simmer 5 minutes, stirring gently, allowing tofu a chance to absorb flavors. Serves 4.

Marinated Tofu Blocks

12 blocks of tofu, ½" x 1" x 2"

one recipe sweet vinaigrette dressing (see recipe)

Marinate tofu in dressing for 15 minutes. remove tofu from dressing; reserve dressing for later. Lightly coat a cookie sheet with canola oil. Place tofu blocks on cookie sheet. Broil at 400 degrees 4-6 minutes per side, or until browned. Serve topped lightly with dressing. Makes 12.

Tomato Bisque

1 cup skim milk

2 Tablespoons flour

½ cup water

2 large tomatoes, peeled, seeded and chopped

⅓ cup minced onion

¼ teaspoon ground cloves

⅛ teaspoon ground pepper

1 teaspoon salt

2 stalks of celery, chopped

Combine milk and flour in a small mixing bowl. Blend with a fork or whisk until smooth. Set aside.

Combine all ingredients, except milk and flour, in a large saucepan, and cook 15-20 minutes or until water is reduced.

Press through a sieve or food mill. Return to saucepan. Add milk mixture. Bring to a boil, stirring well. Reduce heat and simmer one minute. Serves 2-4.

Vegetable Bouillon

2 quarts water

1 teaspoon salt

1 large onion, chopped

5 stalks celery, chopped

1 ob. carrots, peeled and sliced

6 oz. (one small can) tomato paste

¼ teaspoon pepper

1 Tablespoon lemon juice

Combine ingredients in a large pot. Bring to a boil. Reduce heat and cover. Continue cooking, stirring occasionally, for about 30 minutes, until vegetables are cooked. Allow to cool.

Drain and save liquid as your vegetable bouillon. Refrigerate until ready for use. Vegetables may be saved and used for a side dish.

Vichyssoise

1 cup skim milk

3 Tablespoons flour

2 large potatoes, peeled and cubed

1 cup water

1 teaspoon salt

½ onion, minced (about ⅔ cup)

¼ teaspoon pepper

Combine milk and flour in a mixing bowl. Blend with a fork or whisk until smooth. Set aside.

In a medium sauce pan, combine remaining ingredients. Bring to a boil, reduce heat, cover and simmer 30 minutes or until potatoes are soft.

Add milk mixture. Increase heat, bringing to a boil, stirring often. Reduce heat and simmer one minute, stirring constantly, until the liquid thickens.

Remove from heat, run through a food mill, chill and serve. Serves 2-4.

Grilled Veggie Kabobs

4 metal skewers

one yellow squash, cut into ½-inch slices

1 bell pepper

12 pearl onions

8 cherry tomatoes

olive oil

oregano

8 slices of mozzarella cheese, 1" x 4" x ⅛"

Skewer veggies, brush with olive oil, sprinkle lightly with oregano. Grill over indirect flame for 3-4 minutes, turn and cook for two more minutes. Place in a foil tray, top with cheese slices, cover grill and cook for 2-3 more minutes or until cheese is melted. If need, spoon melted cheese back onto veggies, lightly sprinkle once again with oregano and serve.

Pineapple Yogurt Shake

2 cups chopped fresh pineapple

1 cup skim milk

1 cup plain non-fat yogurt

2 Tablespoons sugar

Combine ingredients in a blender. Blend until smooth. Makes about 1 quart.

Corn and Okra Chowder

1 cup water

1 cup of corn, cut fresh from cob

1 cup fresh chopped okra

1 teaspoon salt

¼ teaspoon Tabasco sauce

1 cup skim milk

2 Tablespoons flour

Place water, corn, okra, salt and Tabasco sauce in a medium saucepan. Bring to a boil, reduce heat, cover and simmer for 20 minutes, stirring occasionally.

Combine milk and flour, blending with a whisk or fork until smooth. Add to okra mixture. bring to a boil, stirring often. Reduce heat and simmer for one minute. Serves 2-4.

Homemade Cherry Soda

2 cups carbonated water

3 Tablespoons cherry concentrate or 3 Tablespoons cherry
syrup (see recipe)

Combine ingredients in a tall glass. Stir well and enjoy.

Peach Shake

1 fresh peach, pit removed and peeled

½ cup skim milk

¾ cup non-fat yogurt

1 Tablespoon sugar

Combine peach and milk in a blender. Blend until smooth.
Gradually add yogurt and sugar. Serves 2.

Spiced Buttermilk

2 cups low-fat buttermilk

2 Tablespoons sugar

¼ teaspoon cinnamon

¼ teaspoon nutmeg

¼ teaspoon allspice

¼ teaspoon ground cloves

Combine ingredients in a blender. Blend until frothy. Serves 2.

MAIN DISHES

Baked Zucchini

2 zucchini squash, sliced

1 quart tomato sauce

4 ounces mozzarella, grated

1 onion, thinly sliced

Preheat oven to 350 degrees. Lightly coat a 13" x 9" cooking pan with canola oil.

Arrange zucchini slices in an even layer across bottom of pan.

Top with sliced ovens, again arranging into an even layer. pour tomato sauce over onions, evenly coating all.

Top with mozzarella. Bake at 350 degrees for 45 minutes. Top with parmesan cheese and serve. Serves 4-6.

Rice Parmesan

2 cups cooked rice

4 ounces fresh grated parmesan

1 egg

½ cup skim milk

½ teaspoon salt

1 teaspoon oregano

Preheat oven to 350 degrees. Lightly coat a small casserole dish with canola oil. Set aside.

Combine ingredients in a mixing bowl. Stir well until all is evenly distributed. pour into casserole dish. Bake at 350 degrees for 30 minutes. Serves 4.

Baked Squash

2 acorn squash

1 large sweet onion, minced

2 Tablespoons margarine

Preheat oven to 350 degrees.

Cut squash into halves and remove seeds. Set aside.

Separate onion into 4 equal portions. Place each portion in the opening of a squash half.

Press onions with a large spoon into the squash cavities. Place ½ Tablespoon margarine on top of onions in each squash. Place squash halves in a baking tray.

Cook for 30 minutes at 350 degrees. Brush liquid from squash centers onto exposed edges, and continue baking for 15 more minutes or until a fork inserted into the exposed edges goes in easily. Serves 4.

Veggie Gumbo

4 stalks celery, chopped

1 onion, minced

½ pound of okra, chopped

1 large potato

1 Tablespoon margarine

3 cups water

2 teaspoons salt

1 boiled egg, chopped

1 tomato, peeled, seeded and chopped

½ teaspoon Tabasco sauce

2 Tablespoons flour

Place celery, onion and okra in a large saucepan. peel potato, cut into chunks and add to saucepan. Add margarine and cook until ingredients are browned.

Add remaining ingredients to saucepan, except flour. Cook for about 20 minutes, or until potatoes are tender. Remove about ½ cup liquid from saucepan.

Cool with 1 cube of ice. Blend in flour, stirring with fork or whisk until smooth. Return gradually to saucepan, stirring well. Bring to a boil, reduce heat and simmer 1-3 minutes, until the desired consistency is reached. Serves 4.

Eggplant Pizza

1 eggplant, thinly sliced (about ¼" to ⅜")

olive oil

one tomato, thinly sliced

8 ounces gruyere cheese, grated

4 ounces mozzarella cheese, grated

oregano

Preheat oven to 350 degrees.

Lightly coast a large cooking pan with olive oil. Place eggplant slices on pan.

Brush slices with olive oil. Sprinkle lightly with oregano. top slices evenly with gruyere. Add one slice of tomato to each. Top evenly with mozzarella. Sprinkle lightly once more with oregano.

Bake at 350 degrees for about 20 minutes, or until cheese has melted.

Tofu and Veggie Casserole

1 cup soy or cow's (skim) milk

2 eggs

1 teaspoon salt

2 cups extra firm tofu, cubed

1 yellow squash, quartered lengthwise and sliced

1 bunch broccoli, chopped (about 1½ cups)

½ cup crumbled blue cheese

Preheat oven to 350 degrees. Lightly coat a 2 quart casserole dish with canola oil. Set aside.

Combine milk, eggs and salt in a medium mixing bowl. Blend well with a whisk or fork until smooth. Set aside.

Place tofu, squash and broccoli in casserole dish. Gently fold until evenly distributed. Pour in milk mixture. Sprinkle blue cheese on top.

Cover and cook at 350 degrees for 45 minutes. Serves 4-6.

Egg and Macaroni Salad

½ pound macaroni

⅓ cup mayonnaise

1 coarsely chopped egg

1 garlic clove, pressed

2 green onions, finely chopped

¼ teaspoon salt

⅛ teaspoon pepper

Prepare macaroni according to package instructions. Drain well, rinsing with cold water. Toss in remaining ingredients. Serve chilled. Serves 2-4.

Rice Chili

1½ cups cooked rice

1½ cups water

1 chopped tomato

1 small can (6 ounces) or ½ recipe tomato paste

1½ teaspoons chili powder

¾ teaspoon salt

1 garlic clove, pressed

grated cheddar or Colby cheese (optional garnish)

minced onions (optional garnish)

Combine ingredients in a medium sauce pan. Bring to a boil, cover and simmer 20 minutes. Serve sprinkled with minced onion and grated cheese.

Garden Pasta

½ pound pasta

½ tomato, chopped

1 cucumber, quartered and sliced

½ Greek salad dressing recipe

Prepare pasta according to package instructions. Drain well, rinsing with cold water. toss in remaining ingredients. Serve chilled. Serves 4.

Eggplant Casserole

1 eggplant

2 pieces bread, cubed (stale is OK

8 ounces gruyere cheese

2 eggs

¼ cup canola oil

¼ cup skim milk

⅛ teaspoon paprika

salt and pepper

Preheat oven to 350 degrees. Lightly coat a 3-quart casserole dish with canola oil. Set aside.

Peel and cube eggplant. Sprinkle lightly with salt and pepper. Toss, sprinkle again, and place in casserole dish. Above eggplant, place bread, then cheese. Set aside.

Combine eggs, oil, milk, paprika and ⅛ teaspoon pepper in a medium bowl. Blend well with whisk or fork. pour gently over cheese.

Cover and cook at 350 degrees for 45 minutes. Serves 4.

Variation: If gruyere cheese is not available, it can be replaced with Swiss cheese.

Green Bean Casserole

¾ pound fresh cut green beans

½ medium onion, sliced

6 stalks celery, chopped

2 slices cubed stale bread

1 cup skim milk

2 eggs

1 teaspoon salt

Preheat oven to 350 degrees. Lightly coat a 2 quart casserole dish with margarine.

Combine beans, onions, celery and bread in casserole dish.

Fold until all is evenly distributed. press down gently with a large spoon until the top is level. Set aside.

Combine milk, eggs and salt in a medium mixing bowl. Blend with a whisk until smooth.

Gently poor milk mixture over ingredients in casserole dish. Tamp down lightly until all is covered in milk and top is level. Bake at 350 degrees for one hour. Serves 4.

Baked Rosemary Shells

8 ounces small pasta shells

1 teaspoon rosemary

½ teaspoon dried oregano

4 ounces mozzarella cheese, grated

1 Tablespoon olive oil

1 cup skim milk

1 egg

Preheat oven to 350 degrees. Lightly coat a 13" x 9" cooking pan with olive oil. Set aside.

Prepare pasta shells according to package directions. After draining, toss with rosemary, oregano, olive oil and cheese. Place mixture in cooking pan. Set aside.

Blend milk and egg. Pour into cooking pan, cover and bake for 30 minutes. Serves 4.

Baked Spinach

ingredients from one creamed spinach recipe (see recipe)

2 eggs

Preheat oven to 350 degrees. Lightly mist a 2 quart casserole dish with canola oil. Set aside.

Prepare onions and spinach as in creamed spinach recipe. Set aside. Combine milk, flour, salt and garlic with the two eggs in a medium mixing bowl. Blend well. Combine ingredients in casserole dish. Cover and bake at 350 degrees for 30 minutes. Serves 4.

Linguine Pesto

8 ounces of linguine noodles

¼ cup olive oil

2 cloves pressed garlic

¼ teaspoon salt

¼ cup pine nuts

1 Tablespoon chopped fresh parsley

½ cup fresh grated parmesan cheese

Prepare linguine according to package instructions. Once drained, fold in remaining ingredients, tossing well until all is evenly distributed.

Serve with additional sprinkles of grated parmesan or Romano cheese, if desired. Serves 2-4.

Broccoli Casserole

½ cup skim milk

1 egg

2 cups chopped broccoli

1 cup chopped carrots

½ cup minced onion

4 ounces grated Swiss cheese

Preheat oven to 350 degrees. Lightly coat a 2 quart casserole dish with canola oil. Combine milk and egg in a large mixing bowl. Stir with a fork or whisk until well blended.

Add remaining ingredients. Fold until all is evenly distributed. Transfer to casserole dish. Bake, covered, at 350 degrees for 45 minutes. Serves 4-6.

ABOUT MEAT RECIPES

Eating any kind of meat can increase your chances of risking an attack of gout. However, your physician or dietitian may allow you to eat smaller portions of meat, possibly skinless white meat chicken or turkey.

If your physician has permitted you to include beef in your diet, it will be to your benefit to prepare a dish that will contain less meat than you normally would have consumed, with the smallest amount of purines possible.

For example, meat that has been boiled will contain fewer purines, and its broth should be discarded. Try a tasty sauce from the "Sauces" section to go with that serving.

Furthermore, the amount of meat can be reduced by adding other ingredients, as in our meatball recipe. This dish results in a normal sized serving, with a smaller amount of meat in that serving.

Chicken Kabob

½ pound chicken breast, cut into 1" chunks

4 metal kabob skewers

½ onion, cut into 1" squares

12 cherry tomatoes

1 bell pepper, cut into 1" squares

barbeque sauce (see recipe)

Arrange all items on skewers. Brush well with barbeque sauce. Grill 2½ minutes per side over a medium flame. Check chicken for doneness. Serve with garlic bread. Serves 2-4.

Pineapple Chicken

uncooked rice

½ pound chicken breast, cut into 1" chunks

¼ cup onion, minced

½ cup water

1 cup crushed pineapple

⅓ cup apple cider vinegar

⅓ cup honey

½ teaspoon salt

1 cup flour

Prepare rice according to directions on package **for two servings**. While rice is cooking:

In a large pan, sauté onion in ¼ cup of the water until the onion is transparent and the water is reduced.

Add remaining ingredients, except chicken and flour, to pan. Coat chicken in flour. When ingredients in pan begin to bubble, add chicken to pan.

Reduce heat to simmer, cover and cook 5-7 minutes, turning at least once. Stir often, checking for consistency of sauce and doneness of chicken.

Serve over rice. Serves 2.

Chicken and Dressing Casserole

one recipe dressing (see recipe)

one pound chicken breast

one recipe Garlic Alfredo Sauce (see recipe)

Lightly coat a 13" x 9" pan with canola oil. Set aside.

Cut chicken into ½-inch cubes. Cook in boiling water for 10 minutes. Drain and set aside.

While chicken is cooking, prepare stuffing and Alfredo sauce. Place prepared stuffing in pan, leaving an open area in the middle.

Place the cooked chicken into the open area. Pour ½ of the Alfredo sauce over the chicken only. Cover and bake at 350 degrees for 30 minutes. Before serving, heat remaining Alfredo sauce, blending with a whisk. Place in a sauce boat and serve over the chicken and dressing. Serves 4-6.

Chicken Curry

1 pound chicken breast, cut into 1-inch chunks

1 quart water

⅓ cup minced onion

1 teaspoon salt

⅛ teaspoon pepper

2 Tablespoons margarine

2 teaspoons curry powder

1½ cups water

⅛ cup flour

Drop chicken chunks into 1 quart of boiling water. Return to a boil, then cook 5 minutes. Drain and discard water.

While chicken is boiling, place onion, salt, pepper, margarine and curry powder in a large skillet. Cook, stirring often, until all is browned.

Add chicken and continue cooking until chicken is lightly browned.

Combine water and flour in a small mixing bowl. Stir with a fork or whisk until smooth. Add to skillet, stirring well. Bring to a boil, reduce heat and simmer until the desired sauce consistency is reached. Serve over rice, sprinkled with paprika. Serves 4.

Baked Chicken Dijon

two 8-ounce chicken breasts

1 egg

2 Tablespoons Dijon mustard

1½ cups Italian breadcrumbs (see recipe)

lemon juice

Lightly mist a large cooking pan with canola oil. Preheat oven to 350 degrees.

Trim any fat from chicken. Slice into ¼" thick medallions. Set aside.

Combine egg and mustard. Blend well with a whisk or fork. Dip one piece of chicken into egg mixture, coating well.

Dip in bread crumbs, turning until well coated. Place in cooking pan. Continue with each piece of chicken until all are coated and in cooking pan.

Bake at 350 degrees for about 15 minutes or until crispy, and chicken is completely done. Sprinkle lightly with lemon juice and serve. Serves 4.

Variation: Serve with slices of lemon and sprinkle individually after serving.

Chicken and Dumplings

1½ quarts water

½ pound chicken breast, cut into ¾" chunks

2 cups skim milk

4 Tablespoons flour

1½ teaspoons salt

½ teaspoon pepper

dough from one recipe dumplings (see recipe)

Bring ½ quart of the water to a boil. Add chicken breast. Boil for 5 minutes or until chicken is fully cooked, whichever is longer.

Drain and discard water. Set chicken aside. Combine remaining 1 quart of water, milk, flour, salt and pepper in a large cooking pot. Blend well with a whisk. Add cooked chicken. Bring to a boil, stirring often. Add dumpling dough ½ teaspoon at a time, cooking to desired consistency, about 3 minutes. Serves 4.

Sweet Barbeque Chicken

two 8-ounce boneless chicken breasts

7 pineapple slices

water

honey

4 slices romaine lettuce

Trim chicken. Slice breasts in half sideways. Place in medium saucepan, top with 3 slices pineapple, cover with water and bring to a boil. Boil for 3 minutes. Drain and discard pineapple and water.

Brush chicken and remaining slices of pineapple with honey. Grill over medium direct flame until browned (check for doneness).

Serve each slice over one slice of pineapple on a slice of romaine lettuce. Serves 4.

Variation: Serve over a small bed of rice.

Chicken Salad

8 ounces boneless chicken breast

½ cup mayonnaise

1 stick celery, chopped (about ½ cup)

1 boiled egg, chopped

¼ teaspoon salt

⅓ cup minced onion

⅛ teaspoon fresh ground pepper

Boil chicken breast, until cooked completely through, in lightly salted water. Drain and discard water. Allow chicken to cool. Chop well and place in a medium mixing bowl. Add remaining ingredients, toss well until all is evenly distributed. Serves 4.

Pot Roast

one 2-3 pound pot roast

one sliced onion

4 whole cloves garlic

1 teaspoon whole peppercorns

2 teaspoons salt

4 cups water

Place ingredients in a slow cooker. Cook 4-6 hours on high or 6-8 hours on low setting. Drain and discard everything except the meat. Serve sliced, topped with browned onions or onion sauce. Serves 6-8.

Sloppy Joes

¼ pound lean ground beef

1½ cups water

1 recipe barbeque sauce (see recipe)

Boil beef in water until cooked through. Drain and discard water.

Add barbeque sauce and cook 2-3 minutes, or until desired consistency is reached. Serve over slices of bread. Makes 4.

Stroganoff

1 pound egg (or eggless) noodles

½ pound lean stew beef

½ medium onion, minced

1½ cups water

2 cloves garlic, pressed

1 teaspoon salt

⅛ teaspoon pepper

1 cup milk

1 cup flour

½ cup sour cream

Prepare noodles according to package instructions.

While noodles are cooking: Slice meat ¼" thick. Cut slices into ¼" strips, no more than 2" in length. pound strips into ⅛" thickness. Drop into a pot of boiling water. Cook for 2-3 minutes or until well browned. Drain (discarding broth) and set aside.

In a large skillet, sauté onion and garlic in ½ cup water until onions are transparent and water is reduced. Add remaining 1 cup of water, milk, salt and pepper. Stir well and increase heat to medium-high until it begins to bubble at a light boil. Press meat pieces into flour, being sure to cover thoroughly and evenly. Add to skillet.

Cook, stirring steadily, until the desired consistency is reached. Remove from heat, stir in sour cream.

Serve over noodles. Serves 4.

Meatballs

1 cup fresh parsley leaves (about ⅓ of a bunch)

½ pound lean ground beef

1 cup cooked rice

2 eggs

1 quart tomato sauce

½ teaspoon salt

½ teaspoon oregano

¼ cup flour

Preheat oven to 350 degrees. Line a 13-inch x 9-inch pan with foil. Set aside.

Chop parsley leaves as finely as possible. Place in a large mixing bowl. Add beef, rice, eggs, ½ cup of the tomato sauce, salt, oregano and flour. Mix by hand until all is evenly distributed. The mixture will feel almost soupy.

Shape into 2-inch balls and place in pan. Bake at 350 degrees for 30-35 minutes or until nicely browned.

Serve covered with pasta and remainder of tomato sauce (heated). Makes about 12 meatballs. Serves 6.

Sauerbraten

3-4 pound pot roast

3 cups water

3 cups apple cider vinegar

1 onion, coarsely chopped or sliced

1 Tablespoon whole peppercorns

⅛ cup sugar

one recipe sour cream sauce

Place ingredients (except sour cream sauce) in a slow cooker. Cook for 4-5 hours on high setting, or 6-8 hours on low setting.

Remove meat from slow cooker and discard remainder (this will be a meat broth that now contains many of the purines that were in the meat).

Slice about ⅜ inch thick, add sour cream sauce and serve. Serves 6-8.

Marinated Flank Steak

1 pound flank steak

½ cup apple cider vinegar

1½ cups water

1 sliced onion

4 cloves garlic, pressed

1 teaspoon fresh ground pepper

one recipe onion sauce (see recipe)

Trim fat from steak.

Marinate overnight (at least 4-6 hours) in vinegar, water, onion, garlic and pepper. Discard used marinade.

Lightly sprinkle with salt and pepper. Grill over a medium direct flame for 4-5 minutes per side. Slice thinly and serve topped with onion sauce.

Serves 4.

Fajitas

1 pound flank steak

2 cloves garlic, pressed

½ cup apple cider vinegar

1½ cups water

1 Tablespoon margarine

1 small onion, thinly sliced

½ red bell pepper, thinly sliced

½ green bell pepper, thinly sliced

8 flour tortillas

optional toppings (see below)

Slice flank steak into ⅛" to ¼" strips. marinate overnight in garlic, vinegar and water. Drain and discard marinade.

Heat a large skillet. Add margarine, onion, bell peppers and steak. Grill to desired doneness.

Serve in separate dishes with tortillas and any desired toppings. To eat, wrap steak and desired toppings in tortilla.

Optional toppings can be any or all of the following: salsa (see recipe) sour cream, grated cheese, guacamole, chopped tomatoes, chopped lettuce. Makes 8 wraps.

Beef Rolls

1 pound flank steak

1 medium onion

1½ cups Italian bread crumbs (see recipe)

1 egg

¼ cup skim milk

¼ cup olive oil

3 cloves garlic, pressed

one recipe onion carrot sauce

Preheat oven to 350 degrees. lightly coat a 13" x 9" baking pan with olive oil.

Cut meat lengthwise into 4 strips of equal width. Pound to 3/16" thickness. Drop in boiling water for about 5 minutes. Drain and discard water. Lay the strips flat. Set aside.

Cut onion in half. Slice one half and set aside. Mince remaining half and place in a medium mixing bowl. Add bread crumbs, egg and milk. Stir well until all is evenly distributed. Set aside.

Combine olive oil and garlic, blending well. Brush steak strips with one half of the garlic mixture. Set aside the remaining garlic mixture.

Divide bread crumb mixture into four equal parts. Spread each part evenly over one strip of flank steak. Roll strips and secure with toothpicks. Brush remaining garlic mixture over tops of tolls. Top with sliced onion.

Cover and bake at 350 degrees for 1½ hours. Remove and discard sliced onions. Top with onion carrot sauce. Serves 4.

Beef and Noodles

1 cup water

½ pound lean ground beef

1 teaspoon salt

⅛ teaspoon pepper

½ pound thin egg (or eggless noodles)

2 cups milk

1 Tablespoon flour

1½ cups water

⅓ cup shredded cheese

Combine beef and one cup water in a large skillet. Bring to a boil. Boil until browned, at least one minute. Drain beef and discard broth. return to skillet. Set aside.

Blend milk with flour, salt and pepper until smooth, Add to skillet along with remaining ingredients. bring to a boil, cover and simmer for 15-20 minutes or until noodles are tender. Serves 4.

SIDES
AND
SALADS

Almond Bread

3 cups flour

½ teaspoon salt

1½ teaspoons baking powder

¾ cup sugar

2 Tablespoons margarine

1 egg

½ cup skim milk

¾ cup finely ground almonds

Preheat oven to 350 degrees.

Lightly coat a 4" x 9" bread pan with margarine. Set aside.

Combine ingredients in a large mixing bowl and blend until evenly distributed. Transfer to bread pan.

Bake at 350 degrees for 35 minutes. the top should brown and split. Remove from oven and cool before serving. Serves 4-6.

Yorkshire Pudding Puffs

4 Tablespoons (12 teaspoons margarine)

2 eggs

½ cup skim milk

1 cup flour

½ cup water

1 teaspoon salt

Before beginning, all ingredients must be room temperature.

Preheat oven to 450 degrees. Place 1 teaspoon of margarine in the bottom of each of 12 muffin tins. Place in 450 degree oven to heat margarine and tray.

While the muffin tray is heating, combine remaining ingredients in mixing bowl. Blend with an electric mixer until bubbles form on top.

Remove muffin tray from oven as soon as margarine begins to sizzle. Immediately pour egg mixture into muffin tins, only about ¼" deep each. Bake at 450 degrees for 15 minutes, until brown and puffy.

Do not open the oven while the puffs are cooking - it could cause them to collapse! Serve immediately. Makes one dozen.

Dressing

½ onion, minced

1 stick celery, chopped finely

1½ cups vegetable bouillon (see recipe)

4 cups cubed bread, stale

Bring onion, celery and bouillon to a boil, reduce heat and simmer 2 minutes. Place bread cubes in a large mixing bowl. Pour bouillon mixture evenly over bread cubes, stirring well with a large spoon.

Variation: If there is no bouillon available, lightly salted water may be used.

Dumplings

¼ teaspoon salt

1 egg, well beaten

½ cup water

2 cups flour

Combine salt, egg and water in a medium mixing bowl. Blend well with a fork. Add flour, blending well. Cover and chill for 20 minutes.

When dough is nearly finished chilling, bring 2 quarts of water to a boil. Drop chilled dough into boiling water by ½ teaspoonfuls. Cook for 2-3 minutes, checking for doneness. Drain and serve. Serves 4.

Serving suggestion: Before, serving, toss with 3 Tablespoons melted margarine and ½ cup grated parmesan cheese, or with garlic Alfredo sauce (see recipe).

Coleslaw

1 head of cabbage, shredded

2 carrots, finely grated

¼ cup apple cider vinegar

½ cup canola oil

2 Tablespoons sugar

½ teaspoon salt

Combine ingredients in a large mixing bowl. Stir well and serve. Serves 10-12.

Browned Onions

one large onion

½ cup water

½ teaspoon salt

Thinly slice onion. Sauté in non-stick skillet, stirring often, until browned. Add water and salt.

Stir well until onions are coated with the browned liquid. Cook, stirring well, until water is reduced. Serve over meat, vegetables or bread.

Italian Bread Crumbs

3 slices stale bread (preferably French or Italian)

2 Tablespoons dried chopped parsley

1½ teaspoons dried oregano

4 Tablespoons shredded parmesan

Combine ingredients in a food processor. Blend for about 30 seconds, or until finely ground. Makes about 2 cups.

Variation: If you have no stale bread and want to prepare this recipe, place bread in a 350 degree oven for 10-15 minutes, or place in the toaster (the oven method seems to yield better results).

Dijon Pasta Salad

8 ounces pasta

½ red and ½ green bell pepper, diced

1 cooked egg, chopped

one recipe onion Dijon sauce (see recipe)

Prepare pasta according to package instructions. Rinse with cold water. Toss remaining ingredients and serve. Serves 2-4.

Waldorf Salad

2 large apples, peeled, cored and cubed

4 stalks celery, cut into ½" pieces

⅓ cup yogurt

2 teaspoons fresh chopped mint

Toss ingredients and serve. Serves 4.

Labni Cheese Salad

1 cup pitted black olives

one labni recipe (see recipe)

4 leaves romaine lettuce

Chop one half of the olives. Blend well with labni in a medium mixing bowl. Serve over romaine lettuce, garnished with remaining olives. Serves 4.

Feta Cheese Salad

4 ounces feta cheese, cut into chunks or crumbled

¼ cup sliced black olives

1 cucumber, sliced

8-10 finely sliced onion rings

1 bell pepper, finely sliced

one recipe Greek salad dressing

Toss well and serve. Serves 4.

Mozzarella Salad

8 ounces of mozzarella cheese cut into ¼" cubes

2 Tablespoons apple cider vinegar

6 Tablespoons canola oil

¼ cup minced onion

1 celery stick, cut into bite size pieces

1 clove garlic, pressed

¼ teaspoon oregano

Toss and serve. Serves 2-4.

Sweet Jicama Salad

4 leaves romaine lettuce

1 jicama, peeled and shredded or julienned

1 recipe sweet vinaigrette dressing

1 cucumber, sliced and quartered

½ red bell pepper, diced

Lay romaine leaves on each of 4 salad dishes. Set aside.

Combine remaining ingredients in a medium mixing bowl. Toss until all is evenly distributed.

Place ¼ of jicama salad on each romaine leaf and serve. Serves 4.

Yogurt Cheese

1 pound plain non-fat yogurt

Drain in cheesecloth overnight. refrigerate. Use as a spread, a base for dips or in recipes in place of cream cheese. Makes about 2 cups.

Labni
(Lebanese Yogurt Cheese)

4 cups plain non-fat yogurt

1 Tablespoon salt

Combine ingredients in a medium mixing bowl. Blend well.

Drain 8-12 hours in cheesecloth or over sturdy paper towels in a colander. Flip and drain for an additional 8-12 hours. If using paper towels and a colander, replace paper towels prior to flipping. Serve with pita bread, oil, chopped onions, tomatoes, cucumbers.

Red Cabbage

one head of red cabbage

2 cups water

½ cup apple cider vinegar

½ cup canola oil

½ cup sugar

Remove core from cabbage. Finely chop remainder. Place in large saucepan. Boil in the water for 15 minutes. Drain. Return to saucepan, add remaining ingredients, stir over heat until sugar is dissolved. Serve warm or cold. Serves 8-10.

Baked Okra

½ pound fresh okra

½ cup Italian bread crumbs (see recipe)

⅛ cup shredded parmesan cheese

Preheat oven to 350 degrees. Lightly coat an 8" x 8" cooking pan with canola oil. Set aside.

Remove ends from Okra. Cut into ½-inch slices, toss with bread crumbs. Sprinkle with parmesan. Bake at 350 degrees for 30 minutes. Serves 3-4.

Creamed Spinach

⅓ cup onions, minced

¾ cup water

1 bunch fresh spinach

½ cup skim milk

1 Tablespoon flour

1 teaspoon salt

1 clove garlic, pressed

Chop spinach, removing coarse stems. Set aside.

In a large saucepan, sauté onions and ¼ cup water until water is reduced. Add spinach and remaining water. Cook until wilted. Drain. Set aside.

Blend milk, flour, salt and garlic. Combine with spinach in saucepan. Bring to a boil, simmer one minute, cool and serve. Serves 4.

SAUCES

Tomato Paste

5 large tomatoes

Chop tomatoes and place in a double boiler. Cook, stirring occasionally, until the tomatoes thicken into paste. This could take a few hours.

Press through a strainer. Makes about ¾ cup. This is a good base for soup, chili and sauces.

Sour Cream Sauce

6 ginger snaps, crumbled

⅜ cup sugar

½ cup apple cider vinegar

½ cup water

½ cup sour cream

Combine all ingredients (except sour cream) in a saucepan. Bring to a boil, stirring often. Reduce heat and simmer one minute. Remove from heat, stir in sour cream and serve.

Tart Relish

1 cucumber, finely chopped (about 1 cup)

2 Tablespoons apple cider vinegar

3 teaspoons sugar

¼ teaspoon salt

Combine ingredients, blend well and serve. makes about 1 cup.

Garlic Alfredo Sauce

1½ cups skim milk

2 Tablespoons flour

1 teaspoon salt

3 cloves pressed garlic

⅛ teaspoon pepper

1 teaspoon dried parsley flakes

optional: ⅛ teaspoon oregano

Combine ingredients in a small saucepan. Blend well with a whisk. heat to boiling, reduce heat and simmer one minute, stirring constantly. Makes about 1½ cups.

Italian Garlic Dressing

⅓ cup apple cider vinegar

⅔ cup canola oil

2 cloves pressed garlic

1½ teaspoons mustard

⅛ teaspoon freshly ground pepper

1 teaspoon dried parsley flakes

Combine ingredients in a cruet or mason jar. Cover and shake until well blended. Serve. makes about 1 cup.

Homemade Margarine

½ cup butter

½ cup canola oil

Combine in blender. Blend for about 30 seconds. Transfer to an airtight container and refrigerate.

Sweet Vinaigrette Dressing

⅛ cup apple cider vinegar

⅜ cup canola oil

1 Tablespoon honey

¼ teaspoon dill weed

Combine ingredients in a cruet or mason jar. Cover and shake until blended. Makes about ½ cup.

Onion Sauce

1¼ cups water

2 Tablespoons flour

½ teaspoon salt

½ cup minced onion

Combine 1 cup of the water with flour and salt in a small mixing bowl. blend with a fork or whisk until smooth. Set aside.

Place onions and remaining water in a saucepan. Cook until water has disappeared.

Continue cooking, stirring constantly, until onions are browned. Add water and flour mixture. Bring to a boil, stirring constantly. Reduce heat and simmer one minute, stirring often. Remove from heat and serve.

Can be served over hot vegetables, meat or toasted bread.

Pico de Gallo

1 large, firm tomato, chopped

1 Tablespoon lime juice

½ medium onion or one small onion, chopped

1 bell pepper, diced

Toss ingredients and serve. Can be used as a dip, topping over rice, tacos, fajitas (see recipe), etc.

Salsa

one Pico de Gallo recipe (see recipe)

1 Tablespoon water

¼ teaspoon Tabasco sauce

Place ingredients in pan. Sauté, stirring often, about 5 minutes or until liquid is reduced and sauce thickens. Serve as a dip, over tacos, fajitas (see recipe), etc.

Variation: to adjust spice flavor, add or decrease Tabasco amount by ⅛ teaspoon.

Onion Dressing

⅓ cup minced onion

¼ cup apple cider vinegar

¾ cup canola oil

1 Tablespoon mayonnaise

½ teaspoon rosemary

Combine ingredients in a cruet or mason jar. seal, shake well and serve.

Onion Dijon Sauce

½ cup mayonnaise

¼ cup Dijon mustard

¼ cup skim milk

½ teaspoon salt

¼ cup minced onion

1 clove garlic, pressed

Combine ingredients in a cruet or mason jar. Shake until well combined and serve.

Onion Carrot Sauce

2 cups sliced carrots

¼ teaspoon salt

1½ cups water

½ onion, thinly sliced

Sauté carrots in a medium skillet until browned. Add salt and 1 cup of water. Cook until water is gone. Add onion, cook until browned, stirring often. Add remaining water. Bring to a boil, reduce heat, simmer one minute and serve. Serves 4.

Greek Salad Dressing

⅓ cup lemon juice

1⅓ cups olive oil

⅛ teaspoon freshly ground pepper

2 pinches salt

Combine ingredients in a cruet or mason jar. Shake until blended and serve.

Horseradish Sauce

½ cup sour cream

1 Tablespoon plus ½ teaspoon ground horseradish

Combine in a small mixing bowl. Blend well. Works great as a sandwich spread, dip or veggie topping.

To adjust flavor: If the sauce is too milk, add ½ teaspoon of horseradish at a time to adjust. If it is too hot, add ¼ cup sour cream

Variation: To make a spicy mayonnaise, use mayonnaise in place of the sour cream.

Barbeque Sauce

1 cup catsup

⅓ cup apple cider vinegar

2 cloves pressed garlic

1 teaspoon honey

2 pinches of salt

pepper to taste

Combine ingredients in a medium saucepan. Bring to a boil, reduce heat and simmer 12-14 minutes, or until sauce reaches desired consistency.

Makes about one cup.

DESSERTS

Cheesecake Chiffon Pie

3 eggs

8 ounces cream cheese

$\frac{1}{2}$ cup sugar

$\frac{1}{2}$ teaspoon vanilla

$\frac{1}{8}$ teaspoon nutmeg

2 pre-baked pie crusts **(see recipe)**

one recipe sour cream topping (see recipe)

Preheat oven to 350 degrees.

Separate eggs. Blend egg whites with an electric mixer until peaked. Set aside.

Combine egg yolks, cream cheese, sugar, vanilla and nutmeg. Blend with electric mixer until smooth. Fold in egg whites, blending well with a whisk.

Place one half of batter into each pie crust. Bake 25 minutes at 350 degrees. Remove from oven. Preheat oven to 475 degrees. Cool pies 30 minutes, then spread one half of sour cream topping onto each pie.

Cook at 475 degrees for 5 minutes. Remove, chill and serve. Makes 2 pies.

Sour Cream Topping

1½ cups sour cream

½ teaspoon vanilla

¼ cup powdered sugar

Combine ingredients in a small mixing bowl. Stir until well blended.

Can be used over pies or cakes.

Pie Crust

2 cups flour

½ teaspoon salt

½ cup margarine

½ cup water

For two pie crusts: Sift flour and salt. Cut margarine into flour mixture with a fork. Continue blending with a fork, while adding water.

Knead with floured hands until dough forms into a ball and is not sticky. Chill for 2 hours. Roll to ⅛" thickness on a floured surface.

Cut to an 11" diameter ring, press into one pie dish. Roll remaining dough to ⅛," then press into second pie dish.

Trim edges and discard remaining dough, if any, or use in muffin tins for miniature pies.

Use a fork to prick dough thoroughly across crust. Bake at 400 degrees for 7-8 minutes. Makes 2 crusts.

To bake a 2-crust pie: place one crust into a pie dish, add prepared filling, top with remaining crust. Crimp with fingers, trim edges and cut several vents along radius of crust, leaving at least ½ inch from center and edges uncut. Bake at 350 degrees for 45 minutes or until well browned and filling begins to bubble.

Apple Pie

3 apples, cored, peeled and chopped

½ cup water

2 Tablespoons margarine

2 Tablespoons lemon juice

⅔ cup sugar

½ teaspoon allspice

½ teaspoon cinnamon

½ teaspoon nutmeg

1 Tablespoon flour

2 uncooked pie shells (see recipe)

Combine apples, water, margarine, lemon juice, sugar, allspice, cinnamon and nutmeg in a medium saucepan.

Bring to a boil, reduce heat and simmer 5 minutes or until apples are tender. Remove ½ cup of apple mixture liquid and place in a small mixing bowl. Add one cube of ice, stirring until melted. Add flour, stirring with a fork or whisk until smooth. Return to sauce pan. Bring to a boil, reduce heat and simmer, stirring constantly, for 1-2 minutes, or until liquid is well thickened.

Place inside one pie crust. Top with remaining pie crust. Crimp with fingers to seal and trim off excess crust.

Ventilate top crust with a knife, cutting at least four vents along radius (leave vent cuts at least ½ inch away from edge and center).

Bake in a 350 degree oven for 45 minutes, or until crust is well browned and filling bubbles. Cool at least 10 minutes before serving. Serves 6-8.

Cherry Sauce

one pound fresh cherries, pitted

⅓ cup sugar

2 Tablespoons butter

⅔ cup water

2 Tablespoons flour

Combine cherries, sugar, butter and water in a medium saucepan. Bring to a boil, reduce heat and simmer for 10 minutes, stirring often.

Remove ½ cup liquid from saucepan, cool with one ice cube. Add flour and blend with a whisk until smooth.

Gradually add cooled mixture back to saucepan, stirring well. Increase heat slightly and continue to cook until sauce reaches desired consistency. Serve warm over yogurt, ice cream or cake.

Sour Cream Icing

½ cup sour cream

⅛ cup sugar

Combine ingredients in a small mixing bowl. Blend well with a fork or whisk. Serve over pie, cake or fruit.

Carrot Cake

1½ cups minced carrots

2 cups flour

1 teaspoon salt

2 teaspoons baking powder

½ cup finely chopped or ground walnuts

⅓ cup brown sugar

1 egg

1 cup skim milk

one recipe sour cream icing

Preheat oven to 350 degrees. Lightly coat a 9" x 4" bread pan with margarine. Set aside.

Combine ingredients, except sour cream icing, in a large mixing bowl. Blend well with an electric mixer. Transfer to bread pan. Bake at 350 degrees for 30 minutes or until a toothpick inserted in the center comes out clean.

Cool completely and top with sour cream icing. Serve warm or chilled.

Gingerbread Cake

2½ cups flour

¼ teaspoon salt

1¾ teaspoons baking powder

2 Tablespoons fresh, finely grated ginger root

6 Tablespoons margarine

2 eggs

½ teaspoon vanilla

½ cup brown sugar

⅛ cup molasses

¼ teaspoon cinnamon

¼ teaspoon nutmeg

¾ cup sour cream

Preheat oven to 350 degrees. lightly coat a round cake pan with margarine. Set aside.

Combine ingredients in a medium mixing bowl. Blend with an electric mixer until batter becomes smooth.

Place batter in cake pan and bake at 350 degrees for 45 minutes or until a toothpick inserted in the center comes out clean.

Almond Cookies

¾ cup sugar

½ cup margarine

⅜ cup water

2 eggs

⅓ cup finely ground almonds

1½ teaspoons cinnamon

3½ cups flour

⅛ teaspoon salt

powdered sugar

Preheat oven to 325 degrees. Lightly coat a cookie sheet with margarine. Set aside.

Combine sugar and margarine in a medium mixing bowl. Blend with an electric mixture until creamy.

Add remaining ingredients (except powdered sugar), one at a time, blending until smooth.

Roll on a floured surface to ½" thickness. Cut into 2" rounds and place on cookie sheet. Bake at 325 degrees for 25 minutes. Cookies should become firm, but will not brown.

Allow to cool, roll in powdered sugar. Store separated by wax paper in cookie tin.

Makes about 20 cookies.

Lemon Pudding

2 cups skim milk

½ cup sugar

¼ cup flour

juice of one lemon (about 3 Tablespoons)

Place milk, sugar and flour in a double boiler. Blend well with a whisk. Cool, stirring constantly, until thickened, about 15 minutes.

Add lemon juice. Continue cooking one minute, stirring constantly. Allow to cool 10 minutes before serving. Serves 4.

Cherry Syrup

one recipe cherry preserves

Prepare recipe as for cherry preserves, but rather than pouring into mason jars, press cherries and syrup through a sieve. Serve warm over ice cream, cake, pie, yogurt, pancakes. Makes about 12 ounces.

Yogurt Cheese Cake

1 recipe yogurt cheese

2 eggs

1 teaspoon vanilla

⅓ cup sugar

one pre-cooked pie crust

one recipe sour cream topping

Preheat oven to 350 degrees.

Combine yogurt cheese, eggs, vanilla and sugar in a medium mixing bowl. Blend with an electric mixer until smooth.

Pour into pie crust and bake at 350 degrees for 30 minutes. Allow to cool completely. Add sour cream topping, chill and serve.

Cherry Cheese Cake

one recipe yogurt cheese cake (except topping)

one recipe cherry sauce

Once cheese cake is cooled, top with cherry sauce, chill and serve. May also be served warm.

Twice Baked Sweet Potatoes

4 sweet potatoes

½ cup packed brown sugar

½ teaspoon nutmeg

¼ teaspoon cloves

¼ teaspoon allspice

½ teaspoon cinnamon

1 egg

Preheat oven to 350 degrees. Lightly coat a 2 quart casserole dish with canola oil. Set aside.

Wrap potatoes in foil. Cook in 350 degree oven for 45 minutes. Allow to cool completely. Remove and discard peels. Place potatoes in a large mixing bowl.

Add remaining ingredients and blend well with an electric mixer.

Place in casserole dish. bake at 350 degrees for 30 minutes. Serve warm or cold.

Cherry Crepes

Filling:

2 cups fresh pitted cherries

½ cup water

1 Tablespoon sugar

¼ teaspoon cinnamon

1 Tablespoon flour

Crepes:

½ cup flour

1½ teaspoons sugar

⅛ teaspoon salt

1 egg, well beaten

½ cup skim milk

2 Tablespoons margarine

one recipe sour cream topping (optional)

To prepare filling: Place cherries in a medium saucepan. Combine water, sugar, cinnamon and flour in a small mixing bowl. Blend with a whisk or spoon until the flour has dissolved. Add to cherries. Bring to a boil, stirring often. reduce heat and simmer, stirring often, for 1 minute. Set aside.

To prepare crepes: Combine all ingredients, except sour cream topping, in a small mixing bowl. Blend with a whisk or electric mixer until smooth.

Pre-heat a crepe pan (or 6-inch beveled non-stick skillet). Lightly coat with ¼ teaspoon margarine, for the first crepe only.

Pour in ¼ of the batter. Swirl to even batter thickness. Flip as soon as batter begins to dry on top.

Cook for 15-30 more seconds and remove crepe from pan. Repeat until all 4 crepes are done.

Spread ¼ of the cherry filling along the diameter of each crepe. Wrap loosely and serve, topped with sour cream topping (optional). Serves 4.

Master Index
Books I thru IV

111

Broccoli salad, II
Broccoli salad, II
Broccoli with plum sauce, II
Browned onions, IV
Burgers, veggie, II
Butter, herb, I
Butter, honey, II
Buttermilk, III
Buttermilk biscuits, III
Buttermilk bread, I
Buttermilk salad dressing, I
Buttermilk, spiced, IV
Butternut squash, baked, I
Cabbage, red, IV
Caesar Italian dressing, II
Caesar salad, I
Cake, applesauce, IV
Cake, blueberry coffee, II
Cake, carrot, IV
Cake, ginger coffee, II
Cake, gingerbread & lemon sauce, I
Cake, gingerbread, IV
Cake, orange, I
Cake, sour cream coffee, IV
Cake, vanilla, I
Candied sweet potatoes, I
Cantaloupe fruit salad, I
Carrot cake, IV
Carrot sauce, onion, IV
Carrots and rice, rosemary, II
Carrots, mint, II
Casserole, quiche, I
Celery ranch salad, III
Chef salad, III
Cheese ball, III
Cheese balls, IV
Cheese bread quick snack, I
Cheese casserole, peasant, IV
Cheese dip, pimiento, I
Cheese grits, IV
Cheese potatoes, III
Cheese puffs, chewy, III
Cheese, roasted, II
Cheese rolls, baked, IV

Cheese salad, II
Cheese salad dressing, bleu, I
Cheese salad, feta, IV
Cheese salad, Labni, IV
Cheese salad, Swiss, II
Cheese sauce, III
Cheese soup, II
Cheese, yogurt, IV
Cheesecake, cherry, IV
Cheesecake chiffon pie, IV
Cheesecake, yogurt, IV
Cherry cheesecake, IV
Cherry crepes, IV
Cherry freeze, I
Cherry ice, wild, I
Cherry ice, wild 2, II
Cherry mousse, III
Cherry muffins, IV
Cherry nut bars, II
Cherry pudding crisp, II
Cherry preserves, IV
Cherry sauce, IV
Cherry sherbet, III
Cherry slush, III
Cherry soda, homemade, IV
Cherry syrup, IV
Cherry tea, apple, I
Cherry topping, whipped, III
Cherry yogurt, frozen, II
Cherry yogurt shake, III
Chicken and dressing casserole, IV
Chicken and dumplings, IV
Chicken curry, IV
Chicken Dijon, baked, IV
Chicken kabob, IV
Chicken, pineapple, IV
Chicken salad, IV
Chicken, sweet barbeque, IV
Chicken with pasta, garlic, I
Chili pepper cornbread, II
Chili, potato, I
Chili, rice, IV
Chili with rice, I
Chilies Rellenos, baked, III

Chowder, corn and okra, IV
Cinnamon Toast, III
Coffee cake, blueberry, II
Coffee cake, ginger, II
Coffee cake, sour cream, IV
Coleslaw, IV
Coleslaw, broccoli, II
Cooked apples, I
Cooked pears, I
Cookie dough crust, III
Cookies, almond, IV
Cooler, Mexican rice, I
Corn and okra chowder, IV
Corn, creamed, I
Corn-pepper fritters, baked, IV
Corn pudding, I
Corn soup, III
Corn, tomato and celery salad, III
Corn tortillas, III
Cornbread, II
Cornbread, chili pepper, II
Cottage cheese pie, III
Cranberry tea, II
Cranberry water, II
Cranberry yogurt, II
Cream cheese, low fat, III
Cream of celery soup, II
Cream sauce, sour, IV
Cream sauce, tomato, I
Creamed corn, I
Creamed spinach, IV
Crepes, cherry, IV
Crisps, almond, I, II
Croutons, II
Crust, cookie dough, III
Crust, pie, III
Crust, pie 2, IV
Cucumber Dill Salad, II
Cucumber salad, I
Cucumber sandwiches, II
Curry, chicken, IV
Curry sauce, light, II
Daiquiri, virgin, I
Deluxe fruit crepes, I

Denver omelet, II
Deviled eggs, I
Dijon dressing, II
Dijon pasta salad, IV
Dill sauce, I
Dip, basil ranch, III
Dip, garlic & herb cream cheese, III
Dip, jalapeño, III
Dip, onion, III
Dip, pimiento cheese, I
Double berry mint sorbet, III
Double orange parfait, III
Dressing, IV
Dressing bleu cheese salad, I
Dressing, blue cheese 1 and 2, III
Dressing, blue cheese vinaigrette, III
Dressing, buttermilk salad, I
Dressing, Dijon, II
Dressing, French, I
Dressing, French 2, III
Dressing, Greek salad, IV
Dressing, honey mustard, I, II
Dressing, Italian, II
Dressing, Italian Caesar, II
Dressing, Italian garlic, IV
Dressing, Italian salad, I
Dressing, lemon, II
Dressing, lemon herb, III
Dressing, onion, IV
Dressing, parmesan, II
Dressing, peppercorn, II
Dressing, sweet vinaigrette, IV
Dumplings, IV
Dumplings, potato, III
Egg and macaroni salad, IV
Egg drop soup, II
Egg salad, II
Egg salad wedges, II
Egg sauce, III
Eggplant casserole, IV
Eggplant Italiano, III
Eggplant parmesan, I
Eggplant pizza, IV
Eggplant, sweet and sour, III

Eggplant with lemon pepper pasta, II
Eggs, I
Eggs, deviled, I
Eggs, parmesan, III
Enchiladas, I
Enchiladas 2, II
Evening tea, I
Fajitas, II
Fajitas 2, IV
Falafel, II
Fancy pecans, I
Feta cheese salad, IV
Fizz, pineapple lime, II
Flan, III
Flank steak, marinated, IV
Float punch, III
Flour tortillas, III
Fluffy pancakes, IV
Freeze, berry yogurt, II
Freeze, cherry, I
French dressing, I
French dressing 2, III
French onion soup, I
French toast, I
French toast, orange, II
Fried plantains, I
Fried meat rice, I
Frozen cherry yogurt, II
Frozen yogurt parfait, strawberry, I
Fruit crepes, deluxe, I
Fruit salad, I
Fruit salad, cantaloupe, I
Fruit, spiced, III
Garden pasta, IV
Garlic Alfredo sauce, IV
Garlic bread, I
Garlic chicken with pasta, I
Garlic dressing, Italian, IV
Garlic and herb cream cheese dip, III
Garlic sauce, II
Garlic soup, III
Garlic potatoes, I
Ginger coffee cake, II
Ginger tea, lemon, I, II

Gingerbread cake & lemon sauce, I
Gingerbread cake, IV
Grape leaves, stuffed, I
Gravy, pepper, III
Greek salad, I
Greek salad dressing, IV
Green bean casserole, IV
Green bean salad, II
Green sauce, Mexican, II
Grilled veggie kabobs, IV
Grits, cheese, IV
Gumbo, veggie, IV
Herb butter, I
Hollandaise sauce, III
Honey butter, II
Honey mustard dressing, I, II
Horseradish sauce, III
Horseradish sauce 2, IV
Hot and sour soup, IV
Hot potato salad, I
Ice, lemon lime, II
Ice milk, vanilla, III
Ice, wild cherry, I
Ice, wild cherry 2, II
Icing, sour cream, IV
Italian bread crumbs, IV
Italian dressing, II
Italian dressing, Caesar, II
Italian garlic dressing, IV
Italian salad dressing, I
Jalapeño dip, III
Jalapeños, stuffed, I
Jalapeños, stuffed 2, I
Jicama salad, sweet, IV
Kabobs, grilled veggie, IV
Labni, IV
Labni cheese salad, IV
Lebanese yogurt cheese (Labni), IV
Lasagna, I
Lemon dressing, II
Lemon herb dressing, III
Lemon ginger tea, I, II
Lemon grass tea, I
Lemon lime ice, II

Lemon pudding, IV
Lemon sauce, I
Lemon slush, III
Lemonade, I
Linguine Dijon, III
Linguine pesto, IV
Macaroni and cheese, baked, III
Macaroni and cheese, spicy, III
Manicotti, I
Manicotti in lemon sauce, vegetable,
III
Margarine, homemade, I, II, III, IV
Margarita, virgin, II
Marinated flank steak, IV
Marinated tofu blocks, IV
Matzoh ball soup, II
Mayonnaise, II
Meat fried rice, I
Meatballs, IV
Meatloaf, I
Melon salad, I
Melon sorbet, III
Mexican green sauce, II
Mexican pancakes, II
Mexican polenta, II
Mexican rice, II
Mexican rice cooler, I
Mexican salsa, II
Mint carrots, II
Moussaka casserole, III
Mousse, cherry, III
Mozzarella salad, IV
Muffins, blueberry, I
Muffins, cherry, IV
Mustard dressing, honey, I, II
No-egg pasta, III
Noodle pudding, apricot date, III
Noodles, beef and, IV
Nutty bars, I
Olive and tomato pasta, II
Olive rolls, III
Olive spread, I
Omelet, Denver, II
Onion broccoli quiche, II

Onion carrot sauce, IV
Onion Dijon sauce, IV
Onion dip, III
Onion dressing, IV
Onion pie, III
Onion sauce, IV
Onion soup, French, I
Onions, browned, IV
Onions, squash and, I
Orange and raisin salad, I
Orange cake, I
Orange French toast, II
Orange lime shake, II
Orange parfait, III
orange punch, I
Orange sauce, III
Orange sherbet, III
Pancakes, apple, IV
Pancakes, basic, II
Pancakes, fluffy, IV
Pancakes, Mexican, II
Pancakes, Potato, I, II
Pancakes, rice flour, II
Parfait, double orange, III
Parmesan dressing, II
Parmesan, eggplant, I
Parmesan, rice, IV
Parsley salad, II
Pasta and celery salad, III
Pasta, eggplant with lemon pepper, II
Pasta, garden, IV
Pasta, garlic chicken with, I
Pasta, olive and tomato, II
Pasta, no-egg, III
Pasta salad, I
Pasta salad 2, II
Pasta salad, ranch, III
Pasta salad, summer, III
Pasta shells, sour cream & onion, III
Pasta, tomato, III
Peach shake, IV
Peach yogurt, II
Peaches and cream, hot, III
Pear boat salad, II

Peasant cheese casserole, IV
Pecans, fancy, I
Pepper Dijon, III
Pepper gravy, III
Peppercorn dressing, II
Peppers, pickled, IV
Pesto, linguine, IV
Pesto sauce, III
Picadillo, III
Pickle relish, sweet, II
Pickled peppers, IV
Pico de Gallo, IV
Pie, apple, IV
Pie, cheesecake chiffon, IV
Pie, cottage cheese, III
Pie crust, III
Pie crust 2, IV
Pie, onion, III
Pie, strawberry rhubarb, III
Pie, sweet potato, I
Pie, vegetable pot, III
Pierogies, II
Pilaf, rice, II
Pimiento cheese dip, I
Pineapple chicken, IV
Pineapple yogurt shake, IV
Pineapple lime fizz, II
Pizza, II
Pizza, eggplant, IV
Pizza sauce, II
Pizza sauce, quick, II
Plantains, fried, I
Plum sauce, broccoli with, II
Polenta, I
Polenta, baked, II
Polenta, Mexican, II
Pot Roast, IV
Potato chili, I
Potato dumplings, III
Potato pancakes, I, II
Potato pie, sweet, I
Potato rolls, crunchy, III
Potato salad, I
Potato salad, hot, I

Potato skins, baked, I
Potatoes au gratin, I
Potatoes, candied sweet, I
Potatoes, cheese, III
Potatoes, garlic, I
Potatoes in onion sauce, III
Potatoes, roasted, II
Potatoes, rosemary, III
Potatoes, twice baked sweet, IV
Preserves, cherry, IV
Pudding, apricot date noodle, III
Pudding, basic vanilla, II
Pudding, corn, I
Pudding crisp, cherry, II
Pudding fluff, rice, II
Pudding, lemon, IV
Pudding puffs, Yorkshire, IV
Pudding, rice, I
Punch, float, III
Punch, orange, I
Quiche casserole, I
Quiche, onion broccoli, II
Quiche, western, IV
Quick pizza sauce, II
Quick snack: cheese bread, I
Quick snack: something on a cracker, I
Quick snack: yogurt for dessert, I
Raisin salad, orange and, I
Ranch pasta salad, III
Red cabbage, IV
Rice chili, IV
Rice cooler, Mexican, I
Rice, creamed, III
Rice flour pancakes, II
Rice, meat fried, I
Rice, Mexican, II
Rice parmesan, IV
Rice pilaf, II
Rice pudding, I
Rice pudding fluff, II
Rice, rosemary carrots and, II
Rice, tomato, III
Roast, pot, IV

Roasted cheese, II
Roasted potatoes, II
Rolls, crunchy potato, III
Rolls, olive, III
Rolls, sandwich, III
Rolls, sweet raisin curry, III
Rosemary carrots and rice, II
Rosemary potatoes, III
Rosemary shells, baked, IV
Salad, antipasto, III
Salad, beet, I
Salad, bell pepper, II
Salad, broccoli, II
Salad, Caesar, I
Salad, cantaloupe fruit, III
Salad, chef, III
Salad, cheese, II
Salad, chicken, IV
Salad, corn, tomato and celery, III
Salad, cucumber, I
Salad, cucumber dill, II
Salad, Dijon pasta, IV
Salad dressing, bleu cheese, I
Salad dressing, buttermilk, I
Salad dressing, French, I
Salad dressing, Italian, I
Salad, egg, II
Salad, egg and macaroni, IV
Salad, feta cheese, IV
Salad, fruit, I
Salad, Greek, I
Salad, green bean, II
Salad, hot potato, I
Salad, Labni cheese, IV
Salad, melon, I
Salad, mozzarella, IV
Salad, orange and raisin, I
Salad, parsley, II
Salad, pasta, I
Salad, pasta 2, II
Salad, pasta and celery, III
Salad, pear boat, II
Salad, potato, I
Salad, ranch pasta, III

Salad, stuffed tomato, I
Salad, stuffed tomato 2, I
Salad, summer pasta, III
Salad, sweet jicama, IV
Salad, Swiss cheese, II
Salad, taco, II
Salad, tomato, III
Salad, tropical fruit, III
Salad, vegetable, II
Salad, Waldorf, IV
Salad wedges, egg, II
Salsa, IV
Salsa, Mexican, II
Sandwich rolls, III
Sandwiches, cucumber, II
Sauce, Alfredo, I, II
Sauce, barbeque, IV
Sauce, cheese, III
Sauce, cherry, IV
Sauce, dill, I
Sauce, egg, III
Sauce, garlic, II
Sauce, garlic Alfredo, IV
Sauce, hollandaise, III
Sauce, horseradish 2, IV
Sauce, lemon, I
Sauce, light curry, II
Sauce, Mexican green, II
Sauce, orange, III
Sauce, pesto, III
Sauce, pizza, II
Sauce, onion, IV
Sauce, onion carrot, IV
Sauce, onion Dijon, IV
Sauce, sour cream, IV
Sauce, tomato cream, I
Sauce, white, II
Sauerbraten, IV
Shake, cherry yogurt, III
Shake, orange, lime, II
Shake, pineapple yogurt, IV
Shake, peach, IV
Sherbet, cherry, III
Sherbet, orange, III

Sherbet, strawberry, III
Sherbet, tart lime, III
Shish kabob, I
Shortcake, strawberry, I
Sloppy Joes, IV
Slush, cherry, III
Slush, lemon, III
Slush, strawberry, III
Slush, wild cherry, III
Soda, homemade cherry, IV
Sorbet, double berry mint, III
Sorbet, melon, III
Soufflé, acorn squash, III
Soup, beet, II
Soup, cheese, II
Soup, corn, III
Soup, cream of celery, II
Soup, egg drop, II
Soup, French onion, I
Soup, garlic, III
Soup, hot and sour, IV
Soup, matzoh ball, II
Soup, potato, I
Soup, tomato, II
Soup, vegetable, I
Sour cream and onion pasta shells, III
Sour cream coffee cake, IV
Sour cream icing, IV
Sour cream sauce, IV
Sour cream topping, IV
Spaetzle, II
Spaghetti squash, II
Spice bars, II
Spiced buttermilk, IV
Spiced fruit, III
Spiced tea, I
Spicy macaroni and cheese, III
Spinach, baked, IV
Spread, olive, I
Squash and onions, I
Squash, baked, IV
Squash, baked butternut, I
Squash, spaghetti, II
Squash puppies, III

Steak, marinated flank, IV
Strawberry fluff, II
Strawberry frozen yogurt parfait, I
Strawberry rhubarb pie, III
Strawberry shortcake, I
Strawberry sherbet, III
Strawberry slush, III
Strawberry yogurt, II
Stroganoff, IV
Stuffed bell peppers, I
Stuffed grape leaves, I
Stuffed jalapeños, I
Stuffed jalapeños 2, I
Stuffed tomato salad, I
Stuffed tomato salad 2, I
Stuffed tomatoes, II
Sweet and sour eggplant, III
Sweet barbeque chicken, IV
Sweet jicama salad, IV
Sweet pickle relish, II
Sweet potato pie, I
Sweet potatoes, candied, I
Sweet potatoes, twice baked, IV
Sweet raisin curry rolls, III
Swiss cheese salad, II
Syrup, cherry, IV
Taco melt wedges, II
Taco salad, II
Tamales, III
Tart lime sherbet, III
Tart relish, IV
Tea, apple cherry, I
Tea, cranberry, II
Tea, evening, I
Tea, lemon ginger, I, II
Tea, lemon grass, I
Tea, spiced, I
Toast, French, I
Tofu and veggie casserole, IV
Tofu, BBQ broiled, IV
Tofu blocks, marinated, IV
Tomato bisque, IV
Tomato cream sauce, I
Tomato pasta, III

Tomato rice, III
Tomato salad, III
Tomato salad, stuffed, I
Tomato salad, stuffed 2, I
Tomato Soup, II
Tomatoes, stuffed, II
Topping, sour cream, IV
Topping, whipped cherry, III
Tortillas, corn, III
Tortillas, flour, III
Tropical fruit salad, III
Tropical rice ring, III
Twice baked sweet potatoes, IV
Vanilla cake, I
Vanilla ice milk, III
Vanilla pudding, basic, II
Vegetable bouillon 2, III
Vegetable bouillon, II, IV
Vegetable manicotti in lemon sauce, III
Vegetable pot pie, III
Vegetable salad, II
Vegetable soup, I
Veggie burgers, II
Veggies, blue cheese over, III
Veggie gumbo, IV
Veggie kabobs, IV
Virgin daiquiri, I
Virgin margarita, II
Vichyssoise, IV
Vinaigrette dressing, sweet, IV
Waffles, Belgian, I

Waldorf salad, IV
Water, cranberry, II
Wedges, egg salad, II
Wedges, taco melt, II
Welsh Rarebit, III
Western quiche, IV
Wild cherry ice, I
Wild cherry ice 2, II
Wild cherry slush, III
White Sauce, II
Yellow squash paprika, III
Yogurt, blackberry, II
Yogurt cheese, IV
Yogurt cheese, Lebanese (Labni), IV
Yogurt, cherry vanilla, III
Yogurt, cranberry, II
Yogurt freeze, berry, II
Yogurt, frozen cherry, II
Yogurt honey nut bars, II
Yogurt, low fat, III
Yogurt parfait, strawberry frozen, I
Yogurt cheesecake, IV
Yogurt, peach, II
Yogurt shake, cherry, III
Yogurt shake, pineapple, IV
Yogurt, spiced vanilla, III
Yogurt, strawberry, II
Yorkshire pudding puffs, IV
Ziti, baked, I
Zucchini, baked, IV
Zucchini pesto, steamed, III
Zucchini rolls, II

Bibliography

The information contained in this book was obtained from the following sources:

Aesoph, Lauri M., *How to Eat Away Arthritis*, Revised and Expanded, 1996 Prentice Hall

Arthritis Foundation, "Gout" brochure, 1999, Arthritis Foundation

Biogen Laboratory Developments, LLC, 3189 W Quail Ln, Gresham, Oregon

Chang, David J., "Of all the ginned joints....," *Patient Care*, March 15, 1996, v. 30, n. 5, p.182 (3)

Choi, Hyon K., M.D., DrPH,; Atkinson, Karen, M.D., M.P.H.; Karlson, Elizabeth W., M.D.; Willett, Walter, M.D., DrP.H.; and Curhan, Gary, M.D., Sc.D.; "Purine-Rich Foods, Dairy and Protein Intake, and the Risk of Gout in Men" *The New England Journal of Medicine*, 350:11, March 11, 2004, pp1093-1103

Choi, Hyon K., MD, DrPH, et al, "Coffee consumption and risk of incident gout in men; a prospective study," *Arthritis and Rheumatism*, Vol. 56, No. 6, June 2007, pp. 2049-2055, DOI 10.1002/art.22712, American College of Rheumatology

Choi, Hyon K., MD, DrPH, "Gout," Rheumatic Disease Clinics of North America, Vol. 32, No. 2, May 2006, pp.255-274

Ellman, Michael, H. M.D., "Treating acute gouty arthritis," *The Journal of Musculoskeletal Medicine*, March 1992, pp.71-74

Emmerson, Bryan T. M.d., PhD, *Getting Rid of Gout*, Second edition, 2003, Oxford University Press, Victoria, Australia

Emmerson, Bryan T. M.D., Ph.D., "The Management of Gout," *The New England Journal of Medicine*, Volume 334 Number 7, February 1996, pp. 445-

451

Flieger, Ken, "Getting to know Gout," *FDA Consumer*, March 1995 v29 n2

Forbes Digital Tool: "Cool-Lay off the sheep heart and smelt, or else," wysiwyg://53/http://www,firves,cin/tool.html/97/sep/0920/side2.htm, June 21, 2000, Forbes.com

Ghadirian, P.; Shatenstein, B.; Verdy, M.; and Hamet, P.: "The influence of dairy products on plasma uric acid in women," Eur J Epidemiol 1995; 11:275-81

Gott, Peter, "Gout may be related to medicines," *The Dominion Post*, April 27, 2001

Harness, R. Angus; Elion, Gertrude B.; Zoellner, Nepomuk, *Purine and Pyrimidine Metabolism in Man VII, Part A: Chemotherapy, ATP Depletion and Gout*, 1991, Plenum Press, pp.3, 139-142, 181, 185-203, 217-221, 227-230, 341-344

Lipetz, Philip, M.D., *The Good Calorie Diet*, 1994, Harper Collins Publishers, pp. 188-189

Margen, Sheldon, M.D., *The Wellness Encyclopedia of Food and Nutrition*, 1992, University of CA at Berkeley, health Letter Associates, pp.91-94, 348-358

Martinez-Maldonado, Manuel, "How to avoid Kidney Stones," *Saturday Evening Post*, Sept. Oct. 1995, v.267, n.5, p.36(3)

MayoClinic.com, Salicylates, http://mayoclinic.com/health/drug-information/DR202515

MotherNature.com Health Encyclopedia, Low-Purine Diet, http://www.mothernature.com/ency/Diet/Low-Purine_Diet.asp, 1998, Health Notes, Inc.

National Institute of Arthritis and Musculoskeletal Skin Diseases, "Questions and Answers About Gout," fact sheet, NIAMS Information Clearinghouse, 1 AMS Circle, Bethesda, MD 20892-3675, USA, (301)495-4484

Pennington, Jean A.T., *Bowes & Church's Food Values of Portions Commonly Used*, Edition 17, 1998 Lippincott-Raven, p.391

Porter, Roy and Fousseau, G.S., *Gout, the Patrician Malady*, 1998 Yale University Press

Pritikin, Nathan, *The Pritikin Promise*, 1983, Simon and Schuster, pp. 110-111

Purine Research Society, 5424 Beech Ave., Bethesda, MD 20814-1730, USA, Website: www.purineresearchsociety.org

Sauber, Colleen M., "Still Painful After All These Years. (gout)," *Harvard Health Letter*, v. 20, n. 8, June 1995, p.6(3)

Saunders, Carol S., "Gout: Applying Current Knowledge," *Patient Care*, v. 32, n. 10, May 30, 1998, p. 125

Souci, S.W.; Fachmann, H.; Kraut; *Food Composition and Nutrition Tables*, CRC Press, Medpharm, Scientific Publishers, Stuttgart, 2000, 6th Revised and Complete Edition

Steyer, Robert, "Arthritis Sufferers Put Up a Spirited Fight Against Chronic Pain," *St. Louis Post-Dispatch*, Feb 14, 1999

Strange, Carolyn J., "Coping with Arthritis in Its Many Forms," *FDA Consumer*, March 1996, pp.17-21

Schwartz, George R. MD, *In Bad Taste; The MSG Symptom Complex*, Health Press, New Mexico, 1999

Talboth, John H; Ut, Ts'al-Fan, M.S., *Gout and Uric Acid Metabolism*, 1976, Stratton Intercontinental Medical Book Corp

TruthinLabeling.org, "Hidden sources of processed free glutamic acid (MSG), http://www.truthinlabeling.org/hiddensources.html

Voijr, F. and Petuely, F. *Lebensmittelchemie y. gerichtl. Chemie*, 1982, Vol. 36: 73

Wolfram, G. and Colling, M., *Z Ernahrungswiss*, 1987, v.26, pp.205-13

Zhang, W. et al, "EULAR Evidence based recommendations for gout," *Ann Rheum Dis* published online 30 May 2006 doi:10/1136 ard.2006.055269

Index

Made in the USA
Monee, IL
11 January 2023

25028332R00075